Medical Conditions Requiring Paleo Diet

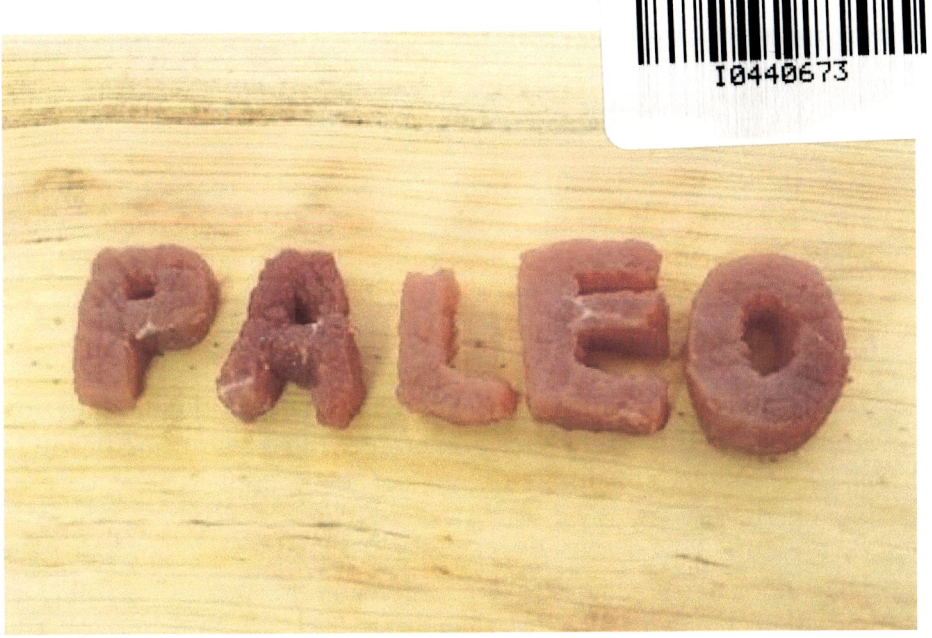

By M. Usman

Health Learning Series

Mendon Cottage Books

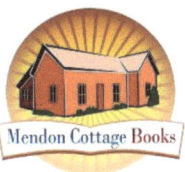

JD-Biz Publishing

Disclaimer

The information is this book is provided for informational purposes only. It is not intended to be used and medical advice or a substitute for proper medical treatment by a qualified health care provider. The information is believed to be accurate as presented based on research by the author.

The contents have not been evaluated by the U.S. Food and Drug Administration or any other Government or Health Organization and the contents in this book are not to be used to treat cure or prevent disease.

The author or publisher are not responsible for the use or safety of any diet, procedure or treatment mentioned in this book. The author or publisher is not responsible for errors or omissions that may exist.

Warning

The Book is for informational purposes only and before taking on any diet, treatment or medical procedure it is recommended to consult with your primary care provider.

Our books are available at

1. Amazon.com

2. Barnes and Noble

3. Itunes

4. Kobo

5. Smashwords

6. Google Play Books

Table of Contents

Introduction: The ancient diet

In the search for the best diet, a theory was presented in the 1980s. The theory reminded humans of their ancestors and the healthy lives they used to live. It blamed the development of modern diseases on our present imperfect diet which it considers a recent innovation as compared to what our bodies have been adapting to, for the major part of history. It says that if we eat the diet of our ancestors, we will return to that healthy state and the diseases of our present time will fade away into non-existence. This is the concept behind paleo diet.

Paleo diet, a modern adaptation of the supposed diet of our ancestors, is claimed to be the solution to the dietary hazards of our time. Can it really provide benefits over our present diet? Can it really be the solution of hazardous diseases that have plagued the modern society? This book discusses the advantages of paleo diet over modern diet relevant to the cure of diseases and assumes the position that indeed, paleo diet can be the solution for the major diseases of our age.

Section One: Knowing Paleo Diet

Diet and nutrition leave a strong impact on our health. The basis of this principle is that what we eat is reflected through our health status. A healthy and balanced diet not only provides you with adequate energy but also improves the quality of life. No one can deny the importance of diet in maintaining a sound health. Certainly our diet has a direct link with our abilities to perform daily activities. For a guaranteed healthy life your diet must be proper and nutritious. No doubt we live in the era of modern civilization. We have the latest technologies, medical facilities, educational and business opportunities. But unfortunately, we have achieved this modernization and civilization at the expense of our health. Every person is running in a race with no destination. Time is running short. Life has become so busy, fast and monotonous. We are so indulged in our daily works and worries that it becomes impossible to give a look at our lifestyles and diet. Our top priority is just to save our time. For this purpose, this modern civilization has provided us with alternatives like junk foods, processed food and ready to eat foods. People now prefer these artificial foods over natural foods like vegetables and fruits. We are happy with our dietary habits being unaware about how these processed foods are damaging our health. The outcomes of these unhealthy foods are health issues like heart diseases, diabetes, obesity, hypertension, Alzheimer's diseases, cancers and bowel diseases. Consumption of high cholesterol and fatty foods has increased the prevalence of heart diseases over the past few years. Similarly, sedentary lifestyle and improper diet are making people obese, increasing the risks of obesity linked disorders like diabetes. No matter, how civilized we are; now the fact is that we are still facing these health issues at a greater rate than in the previous years. This will continue to happen, until and unless we change our eating habits. The need of the hour is to understand that the fault lies within our diet.

After the research of many years, the nutritionists have come forward with the concept of "paleo diet". Paleo diet is a new diet plan for all those people who are concerned about their health. By following this diet plan you can enjoy a better health with the minimum risks of illness. The worldwide success of this diet plan has intrigued many people to learn about the facts of paleo diet. By having a detailed review of paleo diet you will be able to compare the advantages of this diet with your current poor diet.

Paleo diet explained:

The paleo diet is also known by the names "stone age diet", "caveman diet" and "Paleolithic diet". It is based upon diet that our ancestors used to eat 2.5 million years ago. The paleo diet is the modified form of hunters-gatherers diet of Paleolithic era. A comparison of paleo diet with modern diet will help you in assessing the benefits of this ancient diet.

➤ Paleo in Paleolithic era were the habitants of pollution free and natural environment. They were close to nature. They used to eat fresh vegetables, fruits and nuts. But the modern civilization brought many environmental hazards along with it. Improvisation in agricultural techniques has led to many health problems. Use of insecticides and pesticides is a common practice now. These harmful chemicals are absorbed by plants roots, if used carelessly. Their effect persists for a longer time in vegetables and fruits we eat. On the other hand, there was no such usage of harmful chemicals for cultivation in ancient days. That's why our ancestors spend a quality life time.

➤ Researchers are doing work on the evolution of human genome. According to them, 99.5 percent of our genome matches with our ancestors 10,000 years ago. Human physiology is same since the time this world came into existence. Our energy and nutritional requirements haven't changed a bit. But the modern foods have failed to fulfill our energy demands. The foods we are consuming today are mostly processed food. They contain food additives and chemical ingredients to enhance the taste. But unfortunately they are of low nutritional value.

> The people of Paleolithic era were habitual of hunting down and eating fresh lean meat which used to be low in saturated fat content. This explains clearly why our ancestors were at lesser risk of heart diseases. Contrary to this, the junk and fast foods we eat these days are rich in saturated fats. This high content of saturated fats in foods is the main cause of heart diseases.

After this brief discussion we can clearly see the differences between Paleolithic diet and modern diet. The paleo diet is perfect and a balanced diet which ensures a better health. Following the paleo diet plan helps in the management of many chronic diseases like diabetes and hypertension etc.

Dissecting paleo diet: An analysis of its components

Our diet is categorized into two components; macronutrients and micronutrients. A proper ratio of these components is necessary for living a healthy life. Alternation in the intake of either of these essential components might lead to serious health issues. However, the paleo diet claims to have a solution for this. The paleo diet is considered a balanced diet because it contains all the essential components of a diet in the recommended ratio.

Macronutrients of paleo diet:

Macronutrients make up a greater proportion of our body. These are necessary for carrying out various activities in body. Macronutrients are the basic energy yielding molecules. Paleo diet consists of following macronutrients:

Proteins:

Proteins are the most important and recommended macronutrient of paleo diet. The paleo diet suggests increasing the protein intake. Proteins are required for building muscles. High protein diet is also beneficial for people who want to lose weight. High protein intake not only satisfies appetite but also reduces the consumption of carbohydrates. The people of Stone Age were used to getting proteins by hunting the animals and then eating them. High protein food was the secret of their lean body mass. The paleo diet plan, therefore, recommends eating lean meat proteins. Meat should come from those animal sources which are grass fed. Grain fed animals should be avoided because their food contains steroids and synthetic ingredients which are not good for human health. Grass fed beef, sea food, Turkish meat and eggs are the main components of paleo diet. Avoid the usage of processed meat products as they are of low nutritional value.

Fats:

A misconception about fats is that they are harmful for health. But this is not true. Fats are further divided into unsaturated fats and saturated fats. In a normal person the level of saturated level must remain lower than unsaturated fats. Unsaturated fats are essential for the functioning of nervous system. Higher level of saturated fats increases the risks of cardiovascular diseases. Modern diet is, therefore, dangerous for health because it contains high content of saturated fats. The paleo diet focuses on eating lean meat proteins like grass fed beef and lamb because they have low quantities of saturated fats in them. Sea foods are also suggested because they are rich in omega-3 fatty acid. Omega-3 fatty acids are natural anti oxidants which protect the body tissue from inflammation and damage.

Carbohydrates:

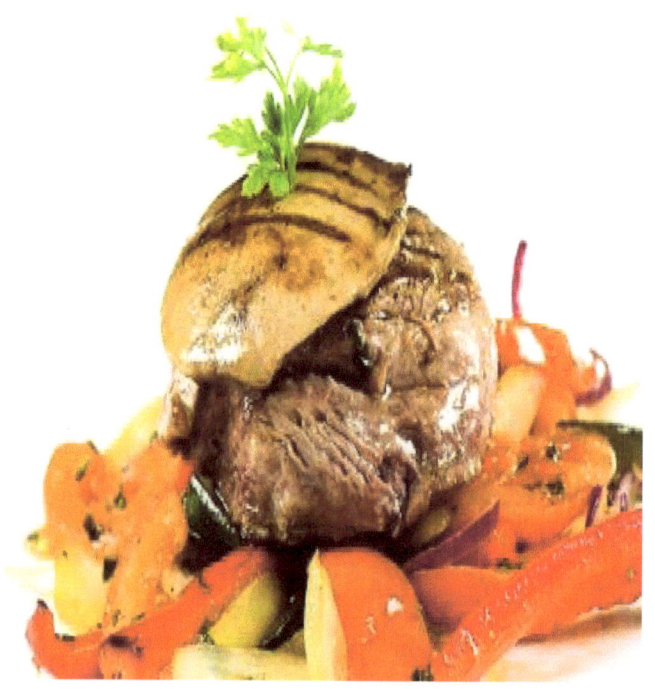

Carbohydrates are the major energy yielding macromolecules but the paleo diet stresses on cutting down the carbohydrates intake. Eating carbohydrate- rich foods elevates the blood sugar level. In response to high glucose level, the production of insulin increases. Insulin converts excess carbohydrates to fats which are then stored into adipose tissues. The undesirable outcomes of carbohydrate consumption are obesity and diabetes.

The paleo diet comprises of foods which have low glycemic index, for example fruits and vegetables. Fruits and vegetables are the richest source of fibers. These fibers not only help in lowering down glucose level in body but also maintaining the normal bowel movements. Avoid taking processed foods like chocolates and bakery products. The foods which are the products of agricultural evolution like legumes, grains and corn are not a part of paleo diet.

Micronutrients of paleo diet:

Vitamins and minerals:

Fruits, vegetables, lean meat proteins and organ meat are the excellent sources of micronutrients. Fish and sea foods contain omega-3 fatty acids which are beneficial for health. Organ meat is the rich source of iron, copper, zinc and selenium which are required for functioning of brain. Green leafy vegetables are enriched with vitamin K, A and calcium. Citrus fruits provide you higher fiber content and vitamin C.

Sodium-potassium ratio:

The foods our ancestors used to eat, millions of years ago, were rich in fruits and raw vegetables. These foods are the excellent sources of potassium. Foods rich in potassium are highly beneficial for health. The concentration of potassium in body should be higher than sodium to prevent the cardiac abnormalities. On the other hand, modern food contains added sodium salt which increases the chances of hypertension and other cardiovascular diseases.

Acid base balance:

Consuming processed food disturbs the acid base balance of body. The contents of modern diet are usually acidic. The acidic diet promotes the development of heart diseases, cancers and renal development. Paleo diet includes alkaline foods, rich in calcium, which neutralize the acidity and bring the acid base balance back to normal.

Foods to eat:

- Lean beef, lamb, Turkish meat, chicken, goat
- Organ meat (liver, brain, kidneys)
- Eggs
- Shellfish, trout, salmon
- Onions, broccoli, Brussels, cucumbers
- Leafy green vegetable like spinach, kale etc
- Nuts and seeds
- Mushrooms
- Dried herbs (parsley, thyme, mint)
- Coconut milk
- Olive oil
- Fish oil
- Fruits like apples, oranges, berries, bananas, mangos

Foods to avoid:

- Legumes

- Grains
- Dairy products
- Artificial sweeteners
- Processed foods
- High sugar foods
- Vegetable oil (corn oil, soybean oil, peanut oil)
- Soft drinks and beverages

Section Two Medical conditions benefitting from paleo diet

Cardiovascular diseases: Heart protecting diet

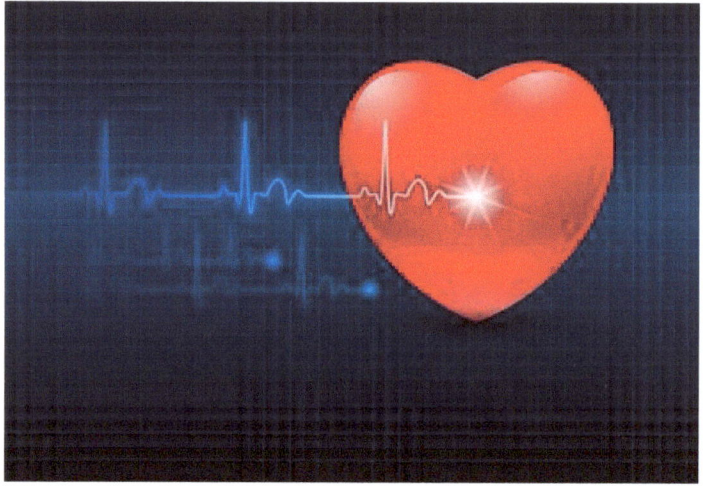

Cardiovascular diseases are increasing day by day. Cardiovascular diseases present with high mortality rate. The factors responsible for cardiovascular diseases include nutritional factors and sedentary lifestyle. All the junk and fast foods we eat have high content of fats and carbohydrates. These foods are the reason for obesity, heart disease, diabetes and hypertension. We have forgotten the importance of exercise in our life. The lack of healthy physical activities and sedentary lifestyles promote the development of heart diseases. We should think about how our ancestors were so fit. They showed no signs of such diseases and lived a healthy and stress-free life. The paleo diet is the modification of caveman diet. The foundations of this diet plan are laid upon the principles of nature. The paleo diet plan relies on all natural foods. There is no place for processed food, synthetic food and artificial food additives in this diet plan. In paleo diet plan all the nutritional factors of nature are in harmony. If we look at the list of foods included in paleo diet, we will find no such food which is harmful for health. The paleo diet is efficacious for many cardiovascular diseases. It helps in curing the following diseases in effective manner:

Coronary heart diseases:

Coronary heart disease usually leads to angina and heart attack. In coronary heart disease the atherosclerotic plaques are formed in the coronary arteries. Coronary arteries are the major vessels which supply oxygenated blood to our heart tissues. Heart muscles require continuous supply of oxygen to keep pumping the blood to whole body. When a person consumes food rich in saturated fats and cholesterol for a longer period of time, the fat and cholesterol level rises in blood. It becomes impossible for our body to metabolize the extra fats.

As a result, the fat and cholesterol molecules start depositing in the walls of coronary arteries. As the time passes, these fatty deposits attract the blood cells towards them. Gradually, an atherosclerotic plaque is formed at this site. These plaques occlude the coronary arteries and compromise the blood flow to heart tissues. The heart muscles get deprived oxygen and become exhausted.

The formation of atherosclerotic plaques is common in people who eat saturated fats and cholesterol-rich foods. Modern diet contains unhealthy fatty food. The cooking oil we use these days has high content of saturated fats and cholesterol. Most of the processed foods we eat are enriched with trans-fatty acids. Trans fatty acids increase the risks of cardiovascular diseases. They are highly hazardous for health.

The paleo diet stresses on consuming lean protein with low content of cholesterol and saturated fats. Grass fed beef, lamb meat, fish and Turkish meat are the excellent sources of proteins along with unsaturated fats. Not all the fats are bad for health. There are some good fats as well i.e. unsaturated fats. Concentration of unsaturated fats must be higher in body than saturated fats to eliminate the risks of heart diseases. The paleo diet contains the foods which are rich in unsaturated fats like nuts and seeds.

The paleo diet encourages you to add fruits and vegetables to your diet. These healthy foods are rich in vitamins and minerals. Formation of atherosclerotic plaque evokes an inflammatory reaction in the coronary arteries. The oxygen-free radicals are formed which cause damage to heart tissues. Vitamins act as anti oxidants which scavenge these toxic radicals. Vitamins confine the inflammation associated with the plaque formation.

The paleo diet contains omega-3 fatty acids in high concentration. Omega-3 fatty acids are highly beneficial for health. They act as anti oxidants. Omega-3 fatty acids have a protective role in preventing heart diseases. That is why paleo diet is highly recommended for patients having heart problems.

Hypertension:

Sometimes the cause behind hypertension or high blood pressure is high blood sugar level. High carbohydrate food can lead to high blood glucose level and insulin resistance. The results of insulin resistance are diabetes and obesity. One way you can control your blood pressure is by reducing carbohydrates and saturated fats in your diet. If you are looking for some proper diet plan for managing your hypertension then you can definitely rely on paleo diet plan. The paleo diet doesn't allow any food which cause high blood pressure.

Obesity: Eat less; get thinner but with more energy...

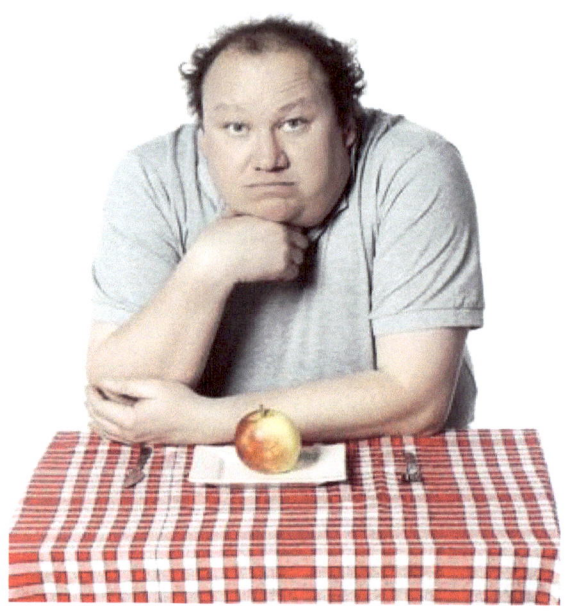

Obesity rate has been constantly increasing over the past few years. The story revolves around carbohydrate intake. The reason behind the higher incidence of obesity is high sugar diet and lack of physical activity. Our lifestyles matter a lot in this perspective. If we compare our lifestyles with the lifestyle of our ancestors in Paleolithic era, we will find hell a lot of difference. They were physically active and strong. Their diet was proper and nutritious. They used to eat fruits, vegetable, meat and nuts. There was no concept of processed and readymade food in those days. This is the reason that they were lean, slim and physically fit.

- Just give a thought to what you are eating today. Your diet is full of junk, fatty and oily foods. You love to eat processed food with the high sugar content. You find these foods to be tasty but remember:

you will have to pay something in return as well. The cost of this poor diet is your precious health. How are you supposed to stay lean and smart when you are eating such foods?

- Carbohydrates are the main culprits behind obesity. If you consume high sugar foods, it raises your blood glucose level and increases your insulin production. Insulin, after utilizing the required glucose promotes the conversion of excess glucose into fats which are then stored in fat tissues of body. This leads to fat accumulation in body and obesity. High insulin makes the muscles resistant to it. Glucose cannot be taken up by muscles. This further accelerates the accumulation of fat in adipose tissues. High insulin also disrupts the balance of another hormone called "leptin". Leptin is a satiety hormone. It is secreted by fat cells of body when fat is accumulated in them. Leptin, in turn, sends signal to brain to stop eating. But this balance gets disturbed in case of high insulin production. Insulin resistance inflames the brain tissue and makes it less responsive to leptin. The leptin production by fat cells keeps on increasing but your brain does not respond to it. The brain doesn't receive any satiety signal and you keep on eating.

- Many obese people want to lose weight but they don't know how to accomplish it. They think that crash diets will them in losing weight. But this is not true. Crash diets and skipping meals might help in losing weight but with some side effects like fatigue and weakness. The answer to these problems is paleo diet. The paleo diet is an effective diet plan for all those people who are keen to lose weight. The paleo diet plan is preferred over other diet plans because of its high nutritional values. The foods components of paleo are in a balanced ratio. The paleo diet plan shifts your diet from high carbohydrate to high protein and low carbohydrate diet. Restricting the carbohydrates in your meals will definitely assist you in losing weight without causing any harm to your health. The paleo diet focuses on calorie intake from proteins rather than carbohydrates. A protein-rich paleo diet will keep you lean and fit.

Diabetes: Too much sweetness, too many problems...

Diabetes is a worldwide disease. The victims of diabetes are increasing in number day by day. It was considered that diabetes has a genetic origin. But now this theory has been improvised as there are many factors which promote the incidence of diabetes. These factors include environmental factors, sedentary lifestyle and modern diet. For understanding the role of diet in diabetes, you must know about whole concept behind this disease.

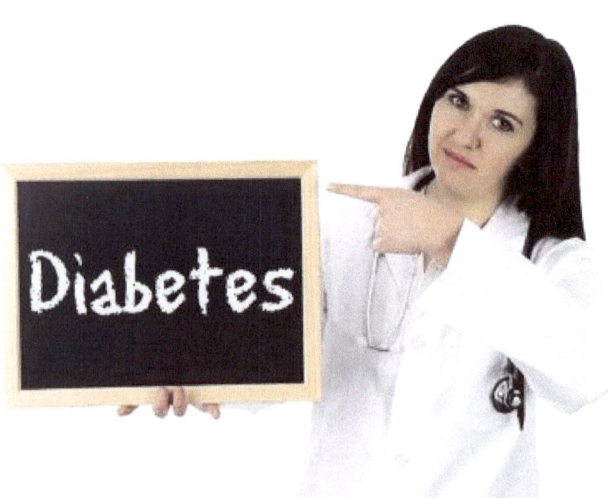

Diabetes is a metabolic disorder in which the body becomes unable to regulate the production of insulin. Insulin the hormone produced by pancreas and secreted in blood. Insulin maintains the level of glucose in blood at normal. Diabetes is classified as; type 1 diabetes and type 2 diabetes. Type 1 diabetes is the autoimmune disorder in which the beta cells of pancreas are destroyed by antibodies, leading to insufficient production of insulin. Type 2 diabetes is quite different from type 1 diabetes. In Type 2 diabetes, the secretion of insulin is higher than normal but the tissues of the body become unresponsive and resistant to insulin.

Normally after taking a carbohydrate-rich meal, the glucose level rises in blood. This alerts the pancreas to increase the production of insulin. Insulin promotes the utilization of glucose by muscles and tissues. After meeting the energy demands of body, the glucose which is present in excess is forced by insulin to enter the muscles where it is converted to glycogen. Glycogen acts as energy reserve. When a person is low on energy, the glycogen is broken down and glucose is released to provide energy. But the modern diet disturbs this normal balance of insulin and increases the risks of Type 2 diabetes in the following ways:

- Modern diet comprises of high sugar foods. These foods elevate the glucose level above normal. In response to this, the insulin production increase. But the repeated intake of carbohydrate-rich food and physical inactivity leads to the constant rise in insulin level. After a certain period of time, the insulin receptors on muscles start degrading. The muscles stop responding to insulin. This phenomenon is called as "insulin resistance". Extra glucose is now unable to enter the muscles.

• The blood glucose level remains high and this keeps on stimulating insulin production. Elevated glucose level is highly dangerous for health. Glucose damages the vital organs of body and starts the inflammatory reaction in whole body. To keep the blood sugar level at normal, you need to cut down your carbohydrate intake. The only way to treat Type 2 diabetes is to avoid the high sugar foods. The paleo diet is the most appropriate dietary regimen for the sufferers of type 2 diabetes. The main benefit of paleo diet is its low carbohydrate content. Restricting the sugar consumption will maintain the insulin and glucose level in the body. The muscles will be re-sensitized to insulin and the inflammatory reaction will be stopped. Thus, it is evident from the whole discussion that the paleo diet has great efficacy in the cure of diabetes.

Sleep problems: A soothing diet

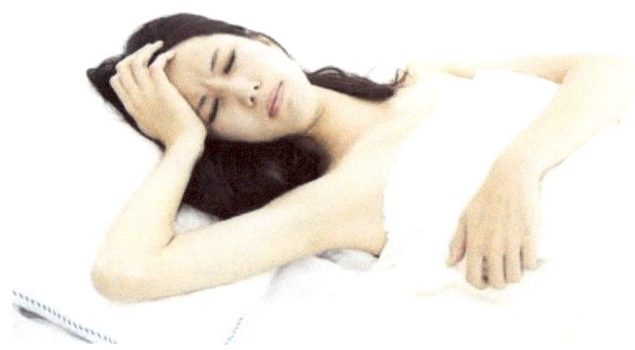

Sleep problem are common these days. Diet has some relation with sleep patterns. A proper sleep of 6-8 hours is necessary for staying healthy and carrying out day to day tasks. Lack of sleep can make you feel anxious, tired, fatigued and restless. Normal sleep and wake cycle is controlled by the release of neurotransmitters from neurons in brain. Any disturbance in the production or release of these neurotransmitters is responsible for changes in normal sleep patterns. Sleep and wake cycle is co related with stress level and dietary habits. Our eating habits not only affect the health but also cause the sleep problems. The increasing trend of sleep problems is associated with the consumption of processed foods, high sugar foods and caffeine. These foods act as brain stimulants. They cause a sudden alteration in energy levels and disrupt the normal sleep.

The paleo diet is a recommended diet for people having sleep troubles. The natural contents of this diet are effective in normalizing the sleep patterns. The paleo diet might help to improve the following sleep disorders:

Insomnia:

Insomnia is commonly seen sleep disorder characterized by difficulty in falling asleep. The quality of sleep becomes poor and the person awakens frequently during sleep. Insomnia is of two types:

- Primary insomnia is caused by psychological disorder, anxiety, depression and mental problems. Normal sleep is regulated by inhibitory neurotransmitters (GABA) and excitatory neurotransmitters (dopamine and glycine). A balance between these neurotransmitters is crucial for inducing proper sleep. Sometimes a diet low in carbohydrates is the reason behind abnormal sleep patterns. Low blood glucose level evokes the "fight and flight" response. There is increased production of cortisols and epinephrine which have stimulatory affect on brain cells. By adjusting the carbohydrates intake, the sleep patterns can be improved. The paleo diet plan offers the solution to this problem. This diet contains the adequate level of carbohydrates and maintains the glucose level in blood. The paleo diet suppresses the sudden elevation in the level of epinephrine and prevents the excitation of brain neurons. The overall affect of paleo diet is to calm down the rapid firing of brain neurons which helps in falling asleep quickly. Micronutrients present in paleo diet, especially zinc and magnesium, have got a significant role in promoting sleep.

- Secondary insomnia is the manifestation of some other underlying diseases like diabetes, celiac disease and restless leg syndrome. The paleo diet helps in inducing sleep by treating these diseases. Diabetic patients usually face sleep problems. Paleo diet comprises of food with low glycemic index which helps improve the condition. Restless leg syndrome is caused by deficiency of iron in body. The protein rich paleo diet corrects the iron deficiency and makes it possible for the sufferer to enjoy a good sleep.

Allergies: "I'm totally natural" says paleo diet.

Here come the other adverse effect of modern diet i.e. allergies. Allergy is the natural immune response of body when there is exposure to certain substances which are normally harmless in the environment. Allergy is an auto immune reaction. When an allergic substance enters the body, our body tries to eliminate it by increasing the production of IgE anti bodies. These anti bodies attack mast cells present in blood and promote the release histamine from them. Histamine evokes a generalized inflammatory response in body. Allergy is manifested as coughing, sneezing, pain, swelling and redness.

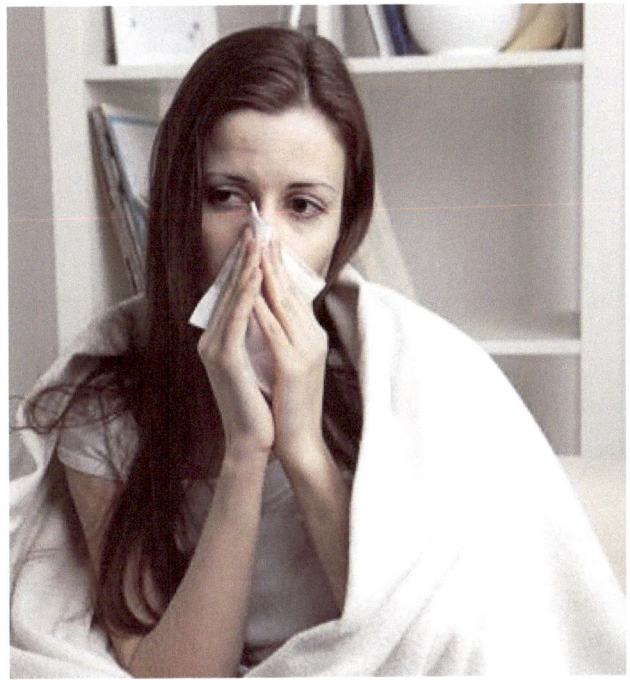

Food allergies are common with modern diet. Chemical ingredients in foods are recognized by the body's immune system as harmful allergens which in turn stimulate the allergic response. Some people are allergic to foods like peanuts, milk, eggs and wheat proteins. The best way to prevent these food allergies is to exclude these foods from your diet.

"I'm totally natural" says paleo diet. This diet is simple and 100 percent natural with no side effects. This naturality of paleo diet and conformity with our genome renders it almost totally non-allergic. The paleo diet is the best diet plan in this regard. Components of paleo diet do not contain any grains, wheat, dairy products and artificial flavors. The paleo diet is based upon the caveman diet. The people of Paleolithic era were more strong and physically fit because what they used to eat was perfectly healthy and balanced. Their diet was composed of lean protein, vegetables, fruits, low carbohydrates foods. This explains that why our ancestors were less affected by allergies, food poisoning and chronic illnesses.

The paleo diet is very effective in curing certain allergic responses. Some of them are discussed here:

Eczema:

Eczema is the allergic response in which the skin becomes inflamed and dry. Rashes and cracks appear on skin. Skin becomes rough, leathery and extremely itchy. Eczema commonly occurs in people who are allergic to certain foods. The foods triggering eczema include soy, peanuts, wheat, milk, eggs. For all those people who are suffering from eczema, the good news is that the paleo diet can help in curing the eczema. The paleo diet restricts the consumption of all allergic foods like milk, peanuts, grains and wheat etc.

Celiac disease:

Celiac disease is the genetic autoimmune disorder of gut. The people with this disorder are allergic to "gluten". Gluten is the protein present in high quantity in wheat, barley and rye. Eating wheat products causes allergic reactions in body characterized by diarrhoea, skin rashes, abdominal discomfort and fatigue. Gluten over activates the body immune system and increases the production of antibodies. These antibodies damage the epithelial lining of small intestine and make the absorption of nutrients difficult through it. However, the paleo diet provides the cure for this problematic situation. The paleo diet is free of gluten rich products like wheat, grains and rye. So, you can get rid of this wheat allergy just by adapting this simple diet plan.

Seasonal allergies:

Seasonal allergies are caused by inhaling airborne pollen and mold spores. Seasonal allergies are common in summer season or when the number of pollen in environment is high. Runny nose, itching eyes, headache and stuffy nose can make your life miserable. Seasonal allergies are triggered by histamine releasing foods like milk, soy, eggs, peanuts, high sugar foods and wheat. Avoiding these foods relieves the allergy symptoms. The paleo diet is the perfect solution for seasonal allergies as it doesn't contain any histamine releasing foods. This superb diet is enriched with vitamins and antioxidants which restrict the inflammation caused by allergic reaction in body.

Skin problems: Bc gone, you rashes!

Acne is the commonest skin problem among all skin troubles. The major reasons for acne are genetic factors, hormonal imbalance and poor diet. Acne affects females more than males. Diet and nutrition are once again important is the prevention of acne. Eating a healthy food might help in improving this condition.

Our skin contains hair follicles in abundance. At the base of these follicles sebaceous or oil glands are present which secrete sebum. Sebum keeps the skin moist and lubricated. Acne erupts when the sebum production by these glands is more than normal. Acne usually affects the face, neck, shoulder and chest region. When the dust particles get trapped within sebum, the pores of follicles are blocked and the pimples are grown in that region. Though acne is under hormonal control yet there are certain foods which trigger the acne formation. Eating oily food, fired food and high sugar foods promotes acne eruption. Let's see how paleo diet is effective in controlling acne problems.

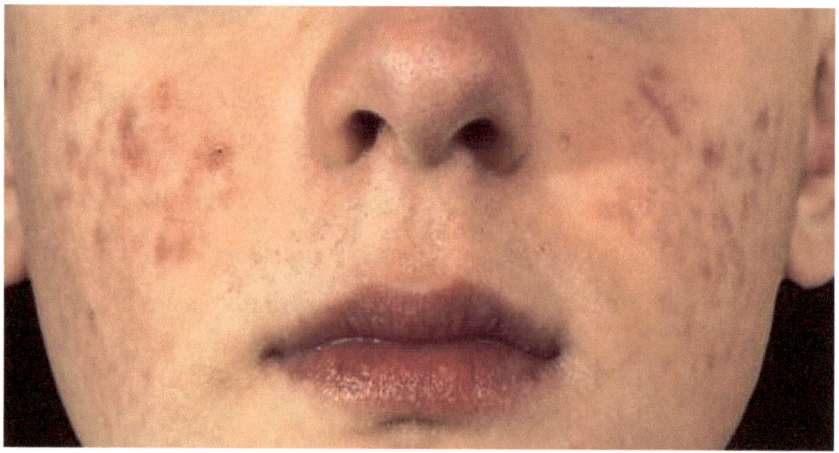

➢ Acne appears on face when the level of androgen hormone is raised in body. Production of androgen hormone is linked with insulin secretion and carbohydrate intake. When you eat carbohydrate rich foods, the blood glucose level rises which in turn stimulates the secretion of insulin from pancreas. High insulin level in blood increases the production of androgens from adrenal glands. These androgens then act on sebaceous gland and enhance sebum secretion. Follow the paleo diet plan if you want to get rid of this troublesome acne, as it includes the foods with low carbohydrate contents. By cutting down sugars in diet, the hormonal level will be adjusted and the acne problem will be resolved.

➢ Another reason for pimples and acne is the poor digestion. The foods we eat today are not good for health. The problems of constipation, bloating and abdominal distention are common with these foods. The paleo diet offers a solution to this problem. Food groups included in paleo diet are fruits and vegetables which are rich in fiber content. Eating these fiber rich foods aids in digestion and helps in relieving constipation. You will see that your acne starts fading once you strictly follow the paleo diet plan.

➤ People are fond of junk foods without knowing how they will affect their health. These foods seem to be tasty and delicious but no one focuses on the chemical ingredients they contain. Food additives and preservatives are the acne causing agents. It is difficult for our body to eliminate or excrete them. That is why paleo diet is considered as the best alternative to this modern diet. The paleo diet contains all natural foods like fruits and vegetables. There are no harmful chemical agents in paleo diet. In fact, the fruits and vegetables are the blood cleansers. They clear off the blood from toxic compounds by detoxifying them. As a result, your skin will start looking younger and glowing.

➤ The paleo diet foods are rich in omega-3 fatty acids. These are the best anti oxidants. Their purpose is to limit the inflammation associated with acne and pimples. Omega-3 fatty acids reduce the redness and swelling around pimples.

➤ Modern diet contains ingredients which are injurious to health. Many women complain of skin problems like wrinkles, freckles and aging marks. No doubt, aging is the natural process but there are many dietary factors which accelerate the aging and wrinkle formation. Improper and unhealthy diet boosts up the formation of toxic oxygen free radicals in body. These radicals contribute to inflammation and skin damage which is manifested as aging marks and wrinkles on skin. For all those women who are worried about their skin problem, here is the best alternative diet plan. The paleo diet is a healthy combination of fruits, vegetables and meat which are rich in all the essential vitamins and minerals. Vitamins promote the growth of skin connective tissue which keeps the skin elastic and taut. Especially, vitamin C is very beneficial for skin and the main source of it is citrus fruits. These vitamins and minerals are natural anti oxidants and are necessary for keeping the skin fresh, firm and wrinkle-free.

Autoimmune diseases: Protecting you from your own self

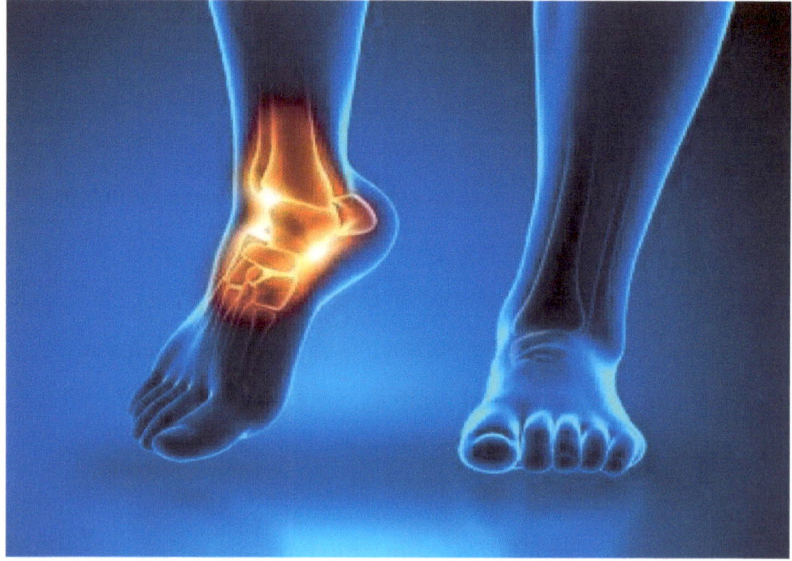

Nature has provided us with the immune system to defend our body against any foreign particles and intruders. Immune system protects us from all kind of infections. When a foreign substance enters the body, the immune system becomes active and produces antibodies which eliminate the foreign particle.

In autoimmune diseases the immune system becomes overactive. The antibodies recognize body's own tissues as antigens or invaders. Thus, antibodies start attacking the healthy tissues of body. The symptoms of autoimmune disorders are inflammation, swelling and redness. The paleo diet is good for many autoimmune diseases like multiple sclerosis, arthritis and lupus erythematosus. The anti oxidants present in paleo diet combat the inflammation and its symptoms. So, paleo diet like some saviour on a knight, seems to reassure you in convincing words: "I shall protect thee from thy own self".

Conclusion

So, it is clear from the discussion in this book that not only does paleo diet improve your health in general but it can also be used to treat and/or avoid specific disease conditions such as heart diseases and can help you live a longer and more comfortable life. It can successfully transport you to an era, where food is still pure and diseases are rare. Health is abundant in this paleolithic era.

Author Bio

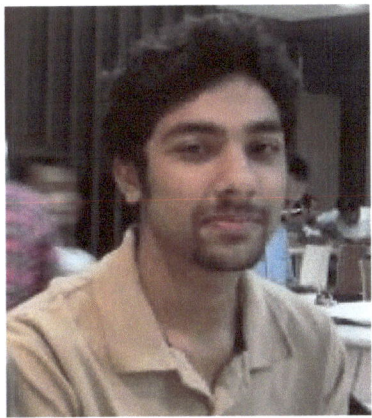

Muhammad Usman is a distinguished medical graduate of Allama iqbal medical college (AIMC). He is a professional writer who has been in the field for more than 4 years. During this time he has produced 10,000+ articles, blogs and eBooks on various niches related to diseases, health, fitness, nutrition and well being. He is a regular contributor to several journals related to medicine and surgery. He is the editor of several journals and newspapers.

Photo Credits

All images licensed by fotolia.com

Medical conditions requiring Paleo diet.

woman and yoga

© *Zdenka Darula - Fotolia.com*

Male patient at the dentist office with a toothache

© *AntonioDiaz - Fotolia.com*

Ankle pain - detail

© *decade3d - Fotolia.com*

she suffers a cold

© *Chepko Danil - Fotolia.com*

gros homme interrogation devant une pomme

© *Laurent Hamels - Fotolia.com*

Basketball

© *Kovalenko Inna - Fotolia.com*

Severe Acne

© *F.C.G. - Fotolia.com*

Checking the glucose level

© *juanrvelasco - Fotolia.com*

Ärztin mit Schild - Diabetes

© *PhotographyByMK - Fotolia.com*

ill woman in bed touching her head

© *Tom Wang - Fotolia.com*

meat and pork liver with sauteed vegetables

© *skyfotostock - Fotolia.com*

Healthy foods in bowl, paleo diet foods, fruits nuts and berries

© *neillockhart - Fotolia.com*

References

1. Walter Voegtlin: The Stone age diet based on in-depth study of Human ecology and diet of man (1975) – CHAPTER 15: A 20th Century Stone age diet (http://www.mitodascalorias.com/wp-content/uploads/2013/06/Voegtlin_1975_The_Stone_Age_Diet.pdf)

2. Wikipedia's definition of Paleolithic diet (http://en.wikipedia.org/wiki/Paleolithic_diet)

3. Walter Voegtlin: The Stone age diet based on in-depth study of Human ecology and diet of man (1975) (http://www.mitodascalorias.com/wp-content/uploads/2013/06/Voegtlin_1975_The_Stone_Age_Diet.pdf)

4. Boyd Eaton, Loren Cordain, Staffan Lindeberg: Evolutionary Health Promotions: A consideration of common counterarguments. December, 2001. (http://thepaleodiet.com/wp-content/uploads/2012/04/Counter-Arguments-Paper.pdf)

5. Boyd Eaton: Paleolithic nutrition – A consideration of its nature and current implications 1985 (http://www.ncbi.nlm.nih.gov/pubmed/2981409?dopt=Abstract)

6. Gary Foster et al. A randomized trial of a Low Carbohydrate diet for Obesity. (http://inspire.stat.ucla.edu/unit_15/NEJM2082.pdf)

7. Staffan Lindeberg et al. Apparent absence of stroke and ischaemic heart disease in a traditional Melanesian island: a clinical study in Kitava.
    (http://onlinelibrary.wiley.com/doi/10.1111/j.1365-2796.1993.tb00986.x/abstract;jsessionid=7F1EEC9B23FCAD9333A2D12078313A4C.d02t01)

8. Loren Cordain and John Friel: The Paleo diet for athletes.
    (http://www.trainingbible.com/pdf/Paleo_for_Athletes_Cliff_Notes.pdf)

9. Dr. John McDougall: The Starch Solution
    (http://www.drmcdougall.com/store_starch_solution.html)

10. Dr. Denis Murphy: People, plants and genes – The Story of Crops and Humanity.
    (http://www.oxfordscholarship.com/view/10.1093/acprof:oso/9780199207145.001.0001/acprof-9780199207145)

11. Katherine Milton: Hunter-gatherer diets – a different perspective
    (http://ajcn.nutrition.org/content/71/3/665.long)

12. Alexander Strohle et al.: Carbohydrates and the diet-atherosclerosis connection--more between earth and heaven. Comment on the article "The atherogenic potential of dietary carbohydrate".
    (http://scholar.qsensei.com/content/1321gb
    http://www.ncbi.nlm.nih.gov/pubmed/16997359)

13. US. News and World Reports 2012 – Best overall diets (http://health.usnews.com/best-diet/best-overall-diets)

Check out some of the other JD-Biz Publishing books

Gardening Series on Amazon

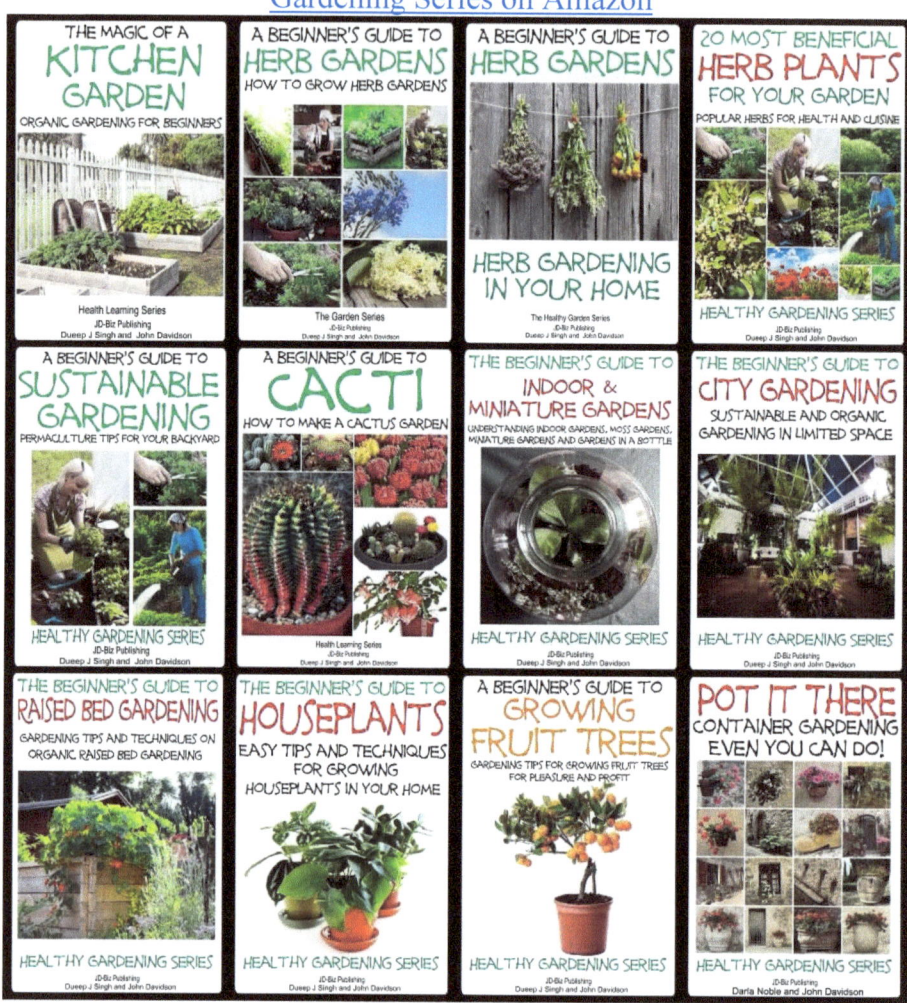

Download Free Books!
http://MendonCottageBooks.com

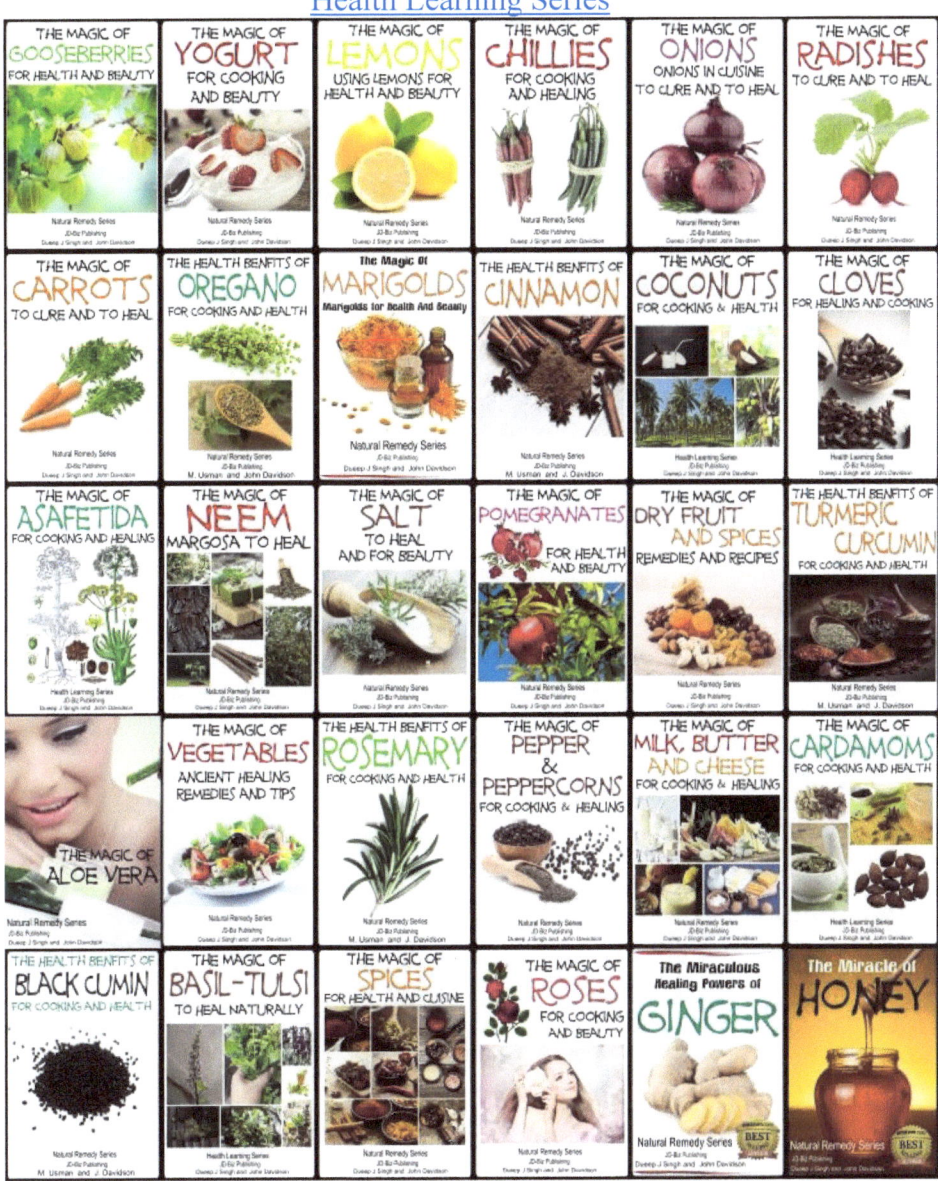

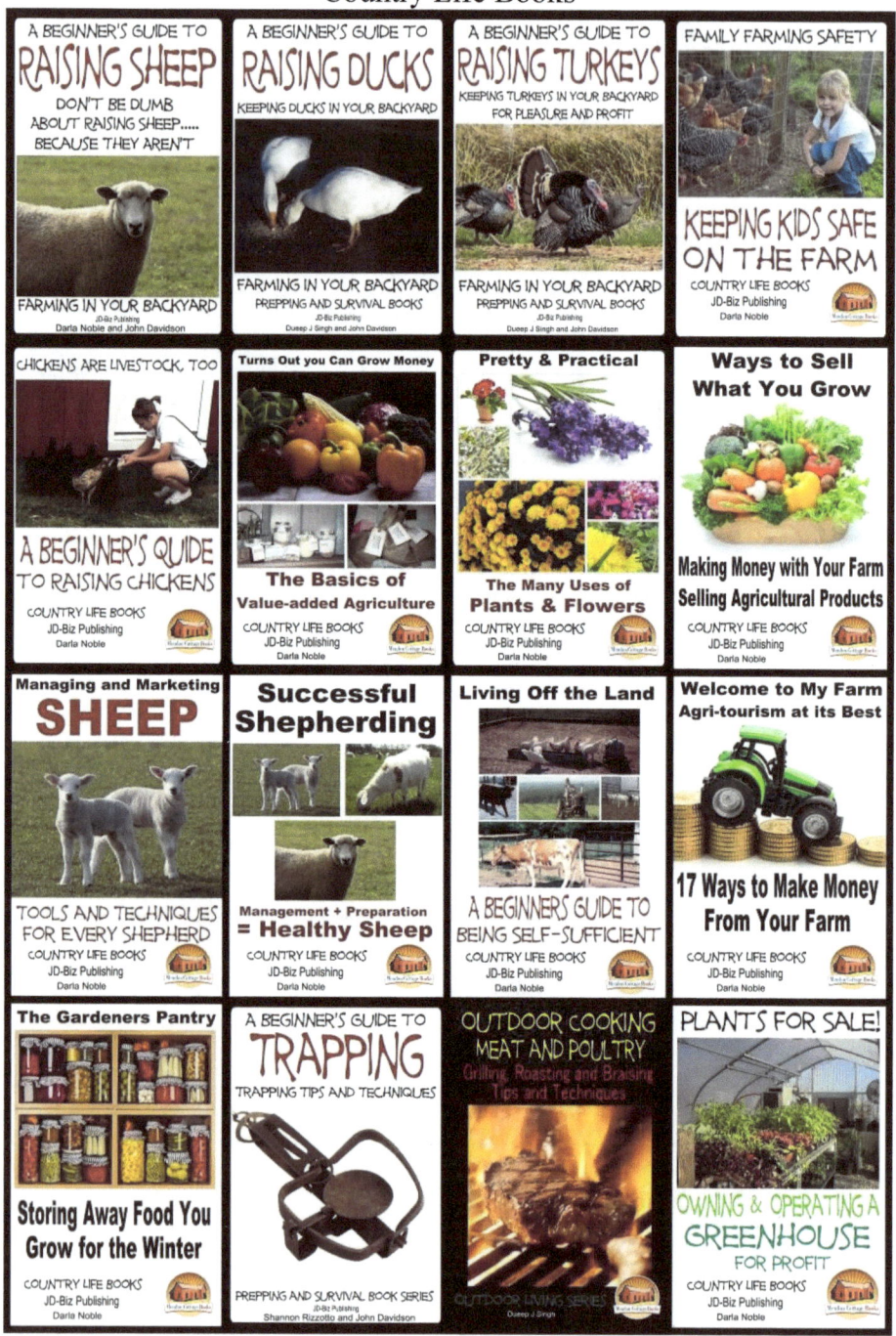

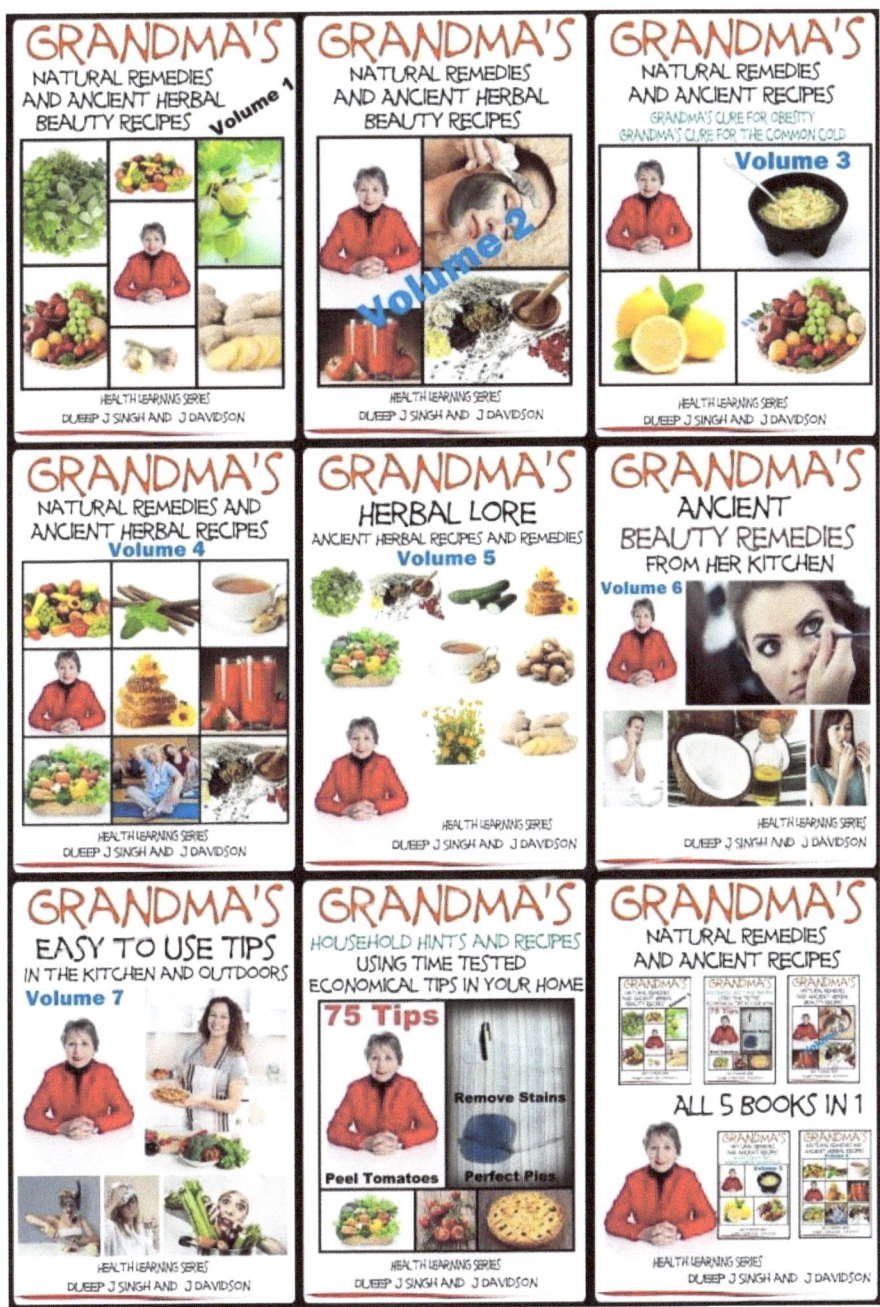

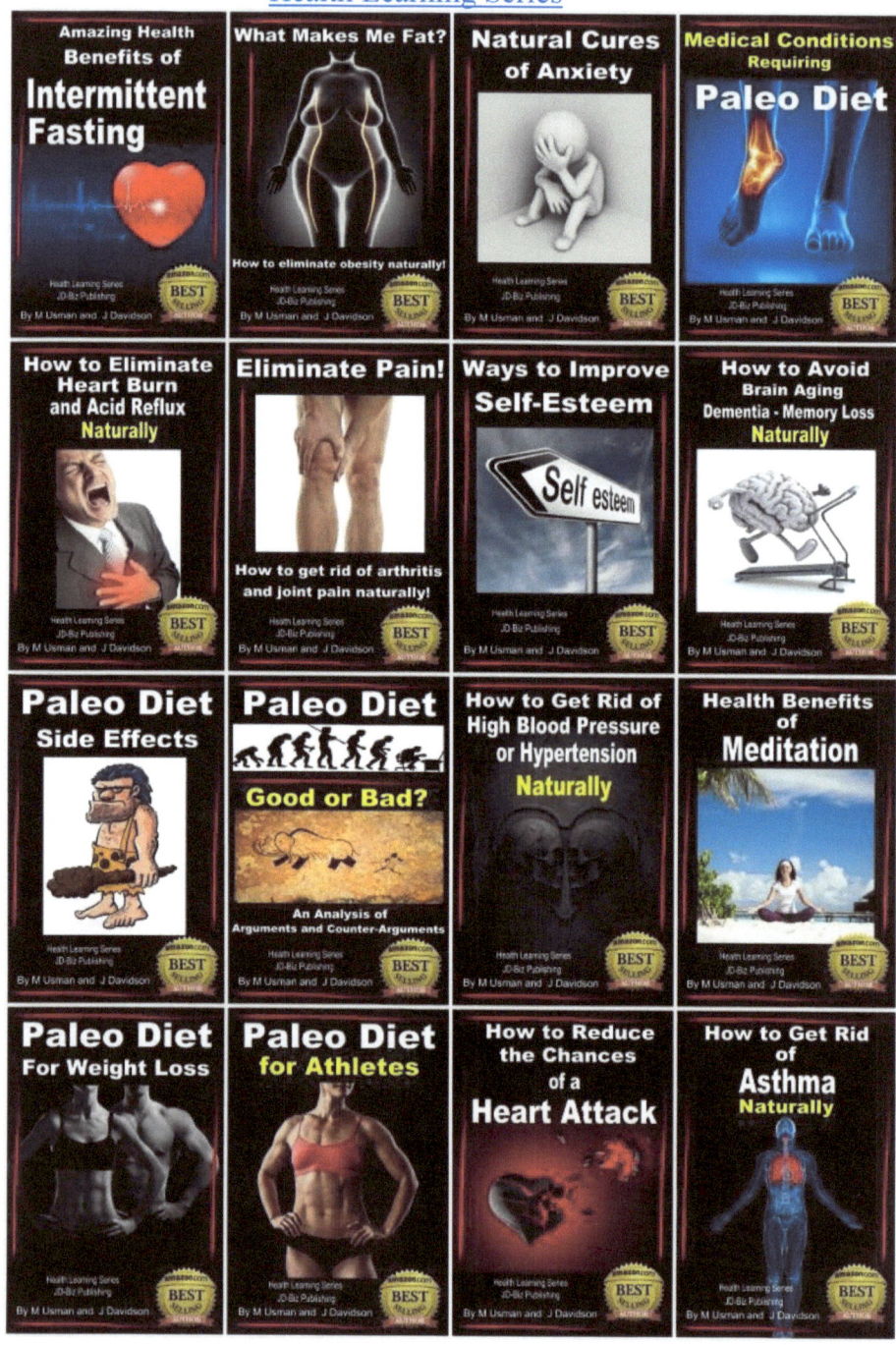

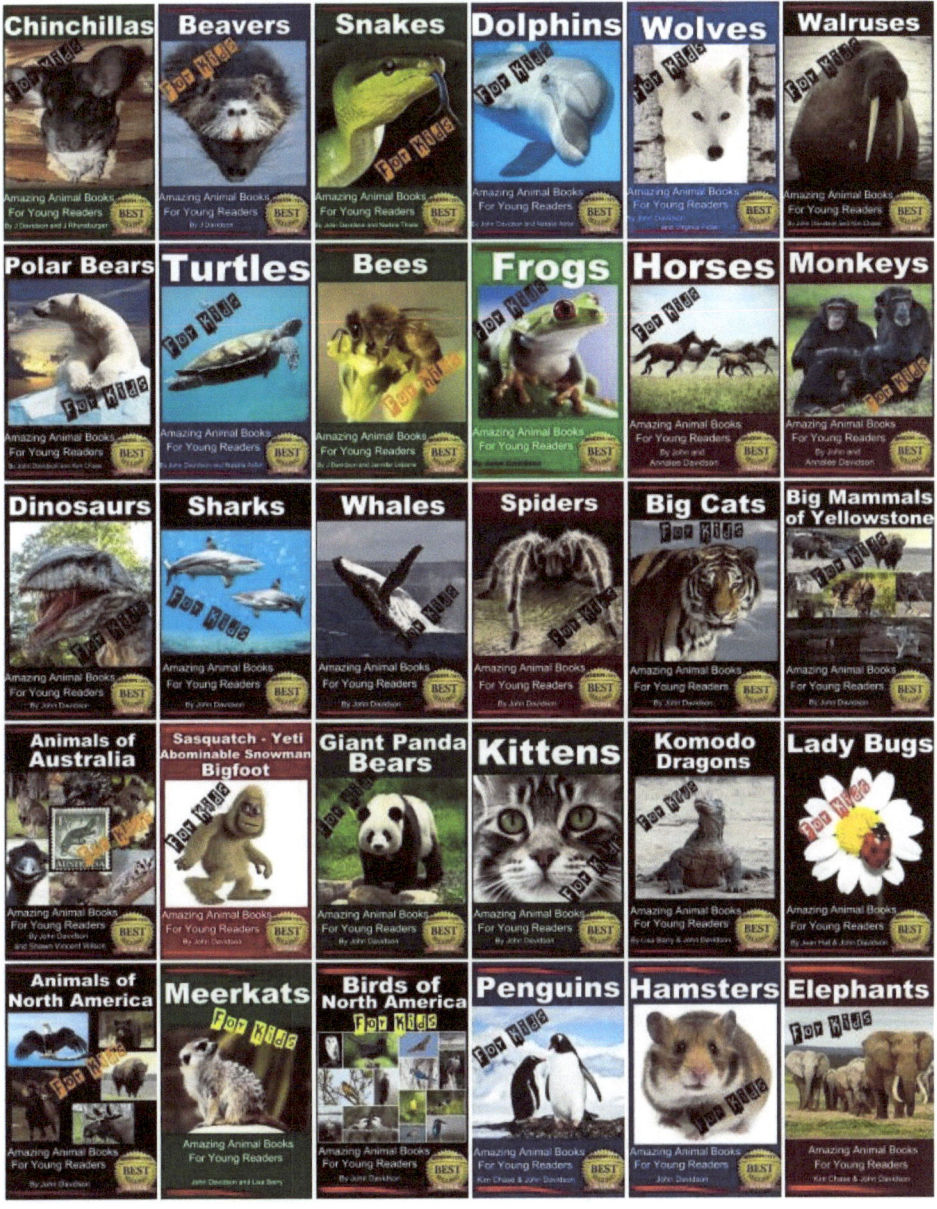

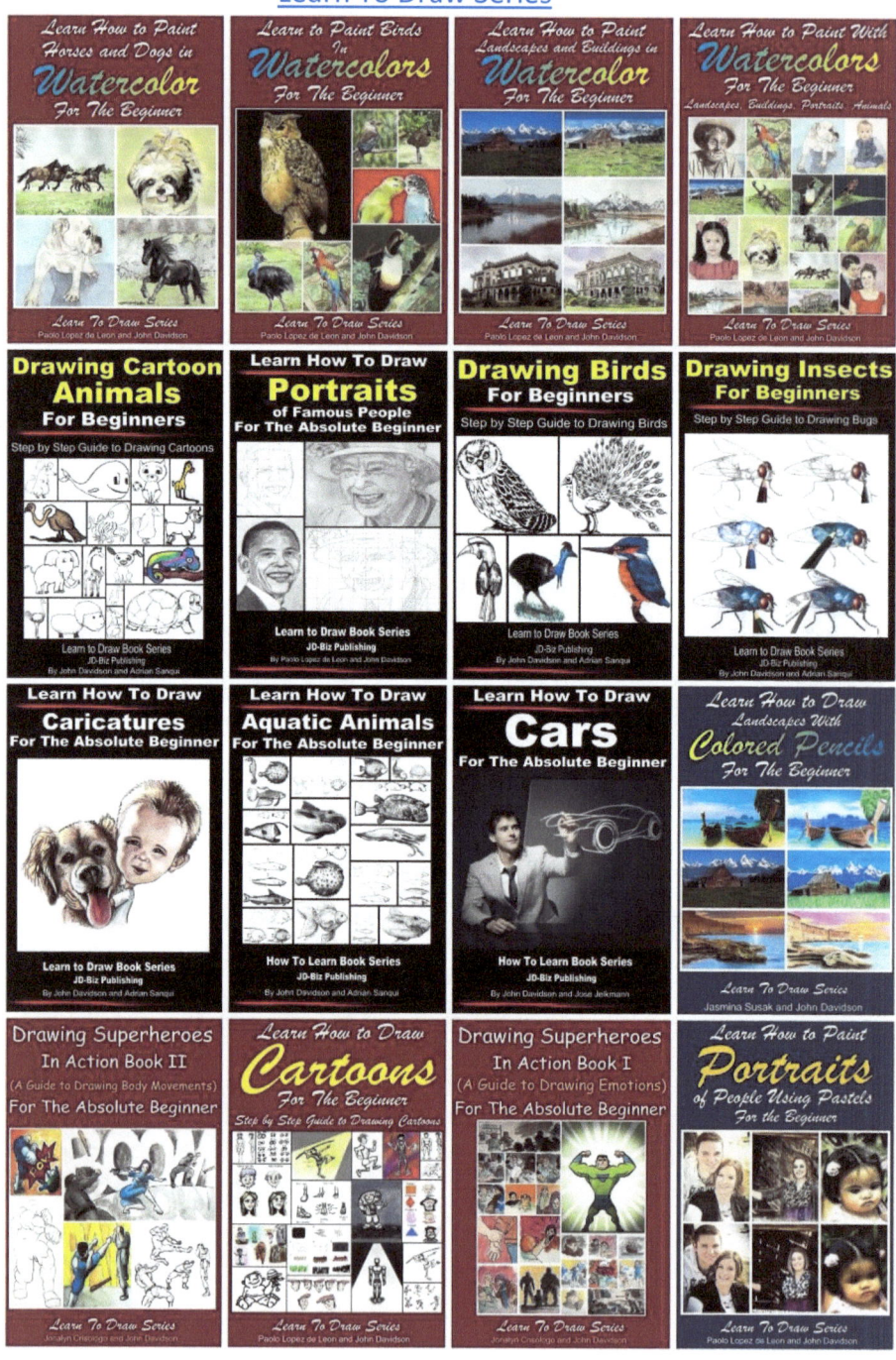

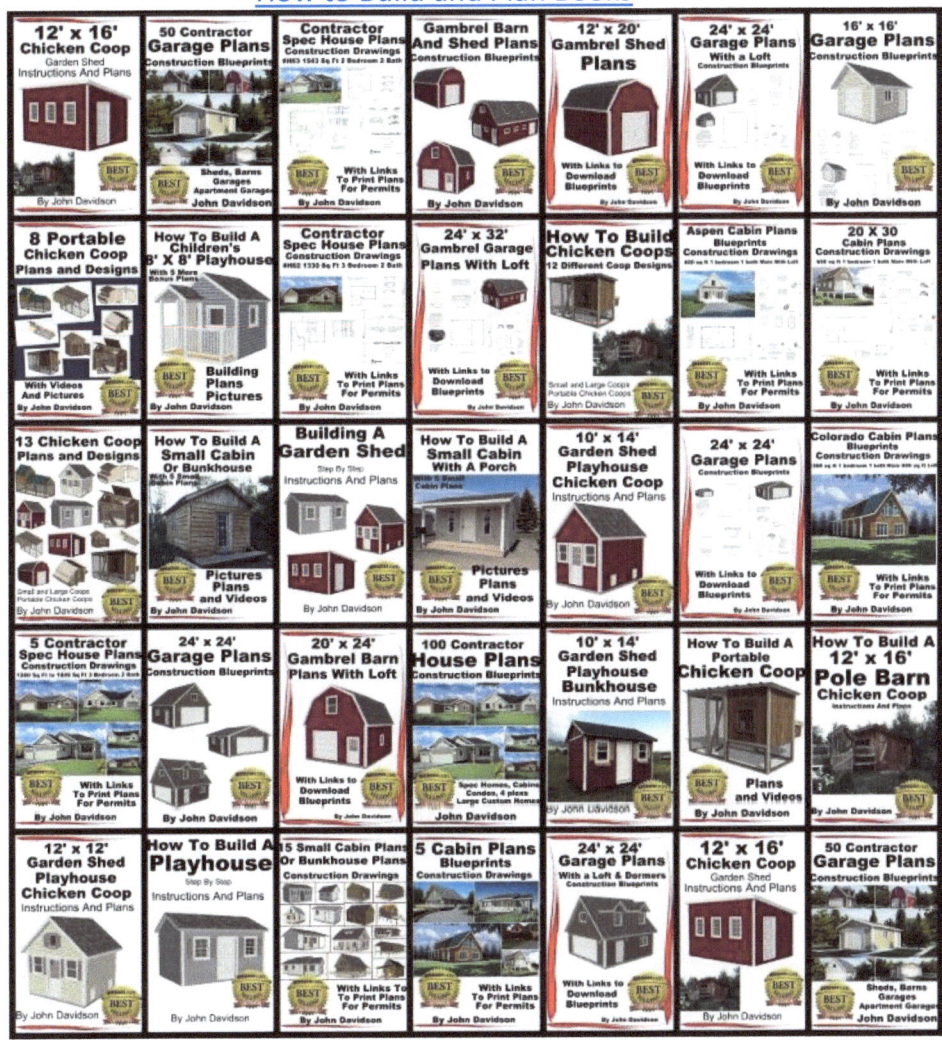

Entrepreneur Book Series

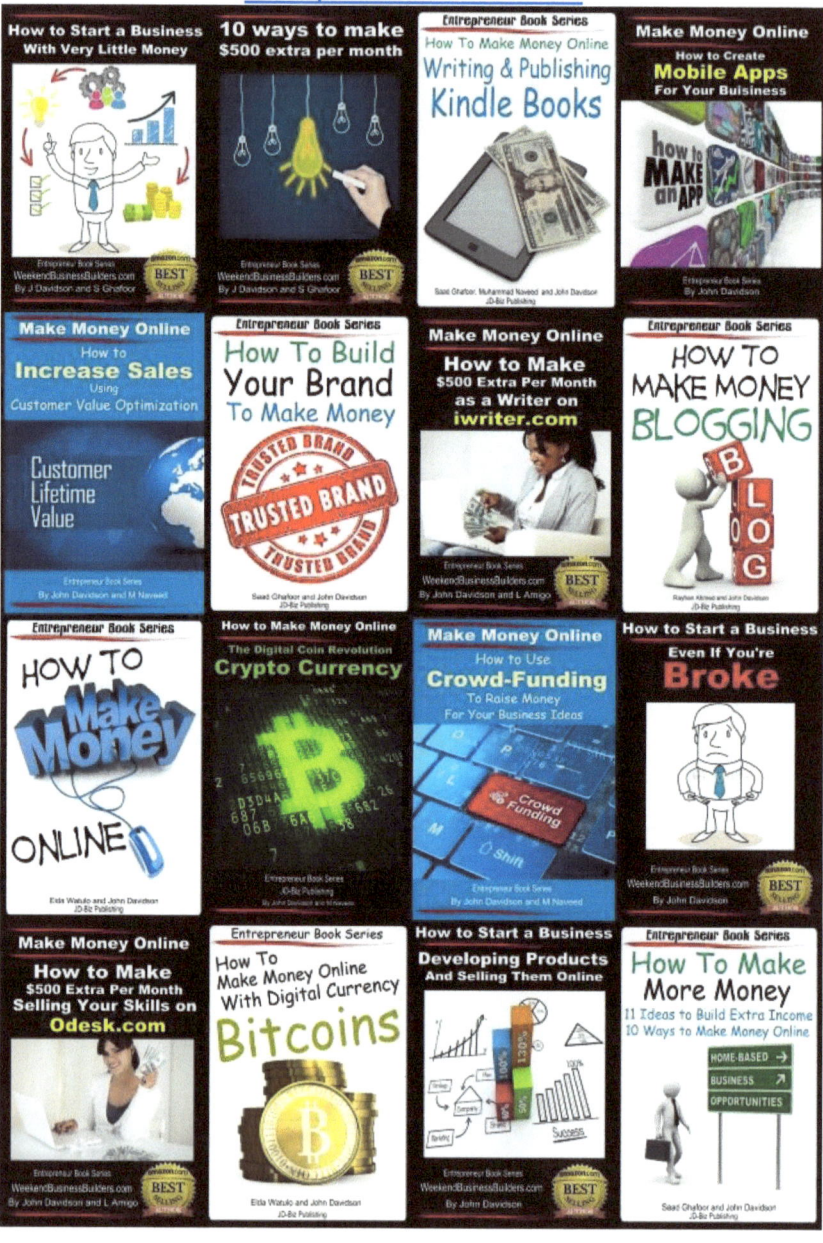

Our books are available at

1. Amazon.com
2. Barnes and Noble
3. Itunes
4. Kobo
5. Smashwords
6. Google Play Books

Download Free Books!
http://MendonCottageBooks.com

Publisher

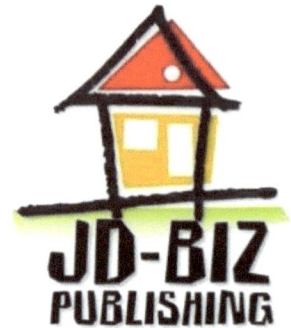

JD-Biz Corp

P O Box 374

Mendon, Utah 84325

http://www.jd-biz.com/

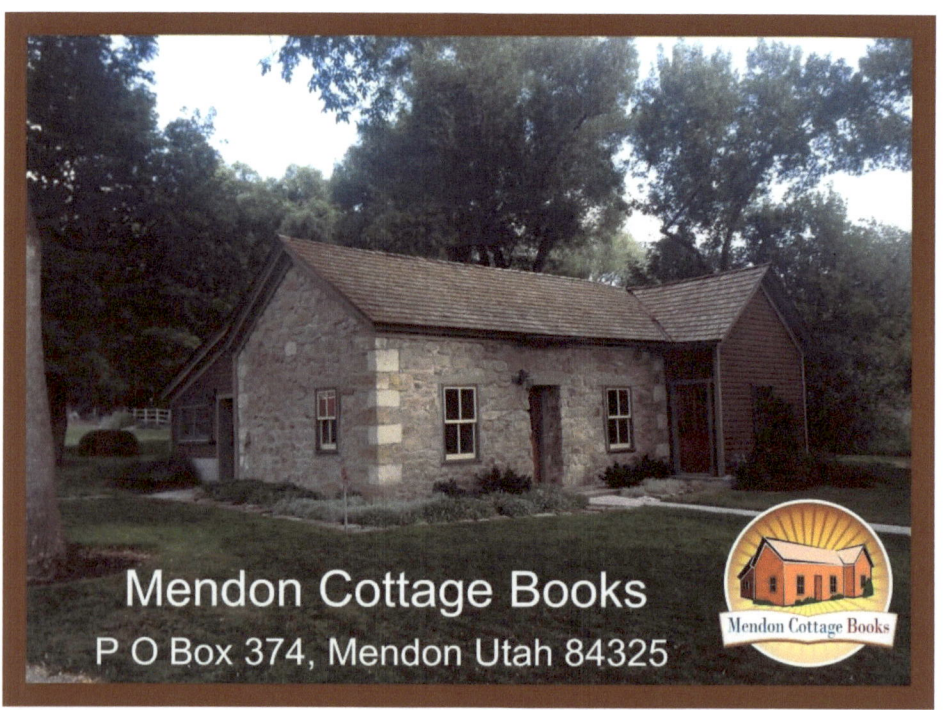

.

www.ingramcontent.com/pod-product-compliance
Lightning Source LLC
Chambersburg PA
CBHW050835290526
45792CB00001B/407